Reverse Diabetes and cause of Diabetes

INTRODUCTION

Welcome to the comprehensive guide on "Reversing Diabetes: Unveiling the Causes and Solutions." In this enlightening eBook, we delve into the intricate web of factors contributing to diabetes while offering practical insights to reverse its course.

Diabetes, a widespread health concern affecting millions, is not merely a condition but a complex interplay of genetic predisposition, lifestyle choices, and environmental influences. This eBook is crafted to empower you with knowledge that goes beyond the surface, exploring the roots of diabetes and its varying forms.

Our journey begins with a thorough exploration of the causes behind diabetes. From genetic markers to sedentary lifestyles, from dietary habits to stress, we unravel the elements that set the stage for diabetes to manifest. Understanding these factors is pivotal in our mission to reverse its effects.

Drawing from the latest research and expert opinions, we then embark on a journey of solutions. Discover a wealth of actionable steps that encompass dietary adjustments, tailored fitness routines, stress management techniques, and more. By addressing the core triggers, we aim to equip you with the tools to potentially halt, and even reverse, the progression of diabetes.

As we navigate through these pages, remember that knowledge is a potent antidote. By comprehending the intricate dance of causes and effects, we empower ourselves to take charge of our health and forge a path towards a diabetes-free future. Join us in this quest to unlock the secrets of reversing diabetes and reclaiming a life of vitality and well-being.

Index

1. Elevate Nutritional Awareness: Embrace a balanced diet rich in whole grains, lean proteins, and vibrant vegetables to regulate blood sugar levels.

2. Prioritise Physical Activity: Engage in regular exercise to improve insulin sensitivity and maintain a healthy weight.

3. Mindful Carbohydrate Management: Monitor carbohydrate intake and choose complex carbs that release energy gradually.

4. Hydration Habits: Stay hydrated to support kidney function and aid in blood sugar control.

5. Strategic Meal Timing: Opt for smaller, frequent meals to prevent spikes and crashes in blood sugar levels.

6. Sugar Scrutiny: Read labels meticulously and reduce added sugars in your diet to curb excessive glucose intake.

7. Portion Control: Be mindful of portion sizes to avoid overeating and maintain steady blood sugar levels.

8. Fibre Incorporation: Include high-fibre foods to regulate digestion, slow glucose absorption, and promote satiety.

9. Healthy Fats Selection: Choose unsaturated fats over saturated ones to support cardiovascular health and insulin sensitivity.

10. Stress Management: Employ relaxation techniques like meditation and deep breathing to lower stress-induced blood sugar spikes.

11. Adequate Sleep Routine: Prioritise sufficient sleep to aid metabolism, hormonal balance, and overall well-being.

12. Regular Monitoring: Keep track of blood sugar levels to identify patterns and adjust your lifestyle accordingly.

13. Weight Management: Achieve and maintain a healthy weight to reduce the risk of insulin resistance.

14. Medically Supervised Plans: Consult medical professionals for personalised guidance, including medications and insulin therapy if needed.

15. Lifestyle Modification: Embrace a holistic approach by combining dietary changes, physical activity, and stress reduction for effective diabetes reversal.

Embarking on this journey armed with these 15 strategies, you can empower yourself to comprehensively address the causes of diabetes while working towards its potential reversal. Remember, your commitment to a healthier lifestyle can pave the way for a brighter, diabetes-free future.

Chapter <1>

Elevate Nutritional Awareness: Embracing Balance for Blood Sugar Regulation

In the intricate tapestry of human health, few factors are as influential as our dietary choices. The foundation of well-being rests upon the sustenance we provide our bodies. This chapter, "Elevate Nutritional Awareness," takes us on a journey through the world of nutrition, guiding us towards a balanced diet that can play a pivotal role in regulating blood sugar levels and potentially aiding in the reversal of diabetes.

The significance of a balanced diet in managing and even reversing diabetes cannot be overstated. Diabetes, a complex metabolic disorder, is intricately intertwined with the foods we consume. By delving into the elements that constitute a balanced diet, we unravel the threads that connect nutrition to blood sugar regulation.

Foundations of Balance: Whole Grains, Lean Proteins, and Vibrant Vegetables

At the heart of this approach lies a trinity of nutritional powerhouses: whole grains, lean proteins, and vibrant vegetables. These components form the backbone of a diet that can help maintain stable blood sugar levels and promote overall health.

Whole Grains: In a world filled with refined carbohydrates, whole grains stand as nutritional champions. Rich in dietary fibre, vitamins, and minerals, whole grains release their energy gradually, preventing rapid spikes in blood sugar. This characteristic is particularly valuable for individuals aiming to regulate their blood sugar levels. Whole grains like quinoa, brown rice, and whole wheat are not only satisfying but also provide sustained energy, reducing the risk of sudden glucose surges.

Lean Proteins: Proteins serve as the building blocks of life, and when chosen wisely, they can be a valuable asset in blood sugar management. Lean protein sources such as poultry, fish, legumes, and tofu offer satiety without causing significant blood sugar fluctuations. Incorporating these protein sources into meals can provide sustained energy while curbing the rapid rise in glucose levels that often follows carbohydrate-heavy meals.

Vibrant Vegetables: The vibrant hues of vegetables are a testament to their nutritional potency. Packed with vitamins, minerals, and antioxidants, vegetables play a dual role in blood sugar regulation. Their fiber content helps slow down digestion, preventing abrupt spikes in blood sugar. Furthermore, antioxidants present in vegetables contribute to overall well-being and potentially mitigate some of the cellular damage associated with diabetes.

The Dance of Balance and Portion Control

While the individual components of a balanced diet offer substantial benefits, the art of portion control ensures their harmonious integration. Portion control is a cornerstone of managing blood sugar levels, as even healthy foods can lead to imbalances if consumed excessively.

Understanding appropriate portion sizes is key to maintaining steady blood sugar levels. Overeating, even with healthy foods, can lead to an influx of glucose that the body struggles to process efficiently. By practicing mindful portion control, we can harness the benefits of a balanced diet while preventing unwanted spikes in blood sugar.

Navigating the Culinary Landscape: Practical Tips

Embarking on the journey of embracing a balanced diet doesn't have to be overwhelming. Here are some practical tips to navigate the culinary landscape and incorporate these principles into your daily life:

1. Meal Planning: Devote time to planning your meals, ensuring a balanced distribution of whole grains, lean proteins, and vegetables. This approach can help you avoid impulsive, less balanced choices.

2. Cooking Techniques: Explore cooking techniques that retain the nutritional integrity of ingredients. Steaming, roasting, and grilling can enhance flavours without compromising the nutritional value.

3. Smart Snacking: Choose smart snacks that align with the principles of balance. Snacking on a handful of nuts or a vegetable-based dip can keep blood sugar levels steady between meals.

4. Mindful Eating: Practise mindful eating by savouring each bite, eating slowly, and paying attention to your body's hunger cues. This approach can prevent overeating and promote better digestion.

5. Label Awareness: Read food labels diligently to identify hidden sugars and make informed choices about the products you consume.

6. Variety Matters: Incorporate a variety of foods into your diet to ensure a broad spectrum of nutrients. Experiment with different grains, proteins, and vegetables to keep meals exciting and nourishing.

In Conclusion: A Path to Wellness

"Embrace a balanced diet rich in whole grains, lean proteins, and vibrant vegetables" is not merely a dietary directive; it's an invitation to transform your relationship with food and harness its potential to positively impact your health. By understanding the significance of these nutritional elements and integrating them into your meals, you can take significant strides towards regulating blood sugar levels and working towards the potential reversal of diabetes. As you embark on this journey of nutritional awareness, remember that small, intentional choices can create a profound ripple effect, fostering a healthier and more vibrant life.

Chapter <2>

Prioritise Physical Activity: Unlocking Wellness through Regular Exercise

In the realm of holistic health, few practices hold as much transformative power as regular physical activity. The chapter "Prioritise Physical Activity" serves as a beacon, illuminating the profound impact that exercise can have on improving insulin sensitivity and cultivating a healthy weight. As we navigate this chapter, we'll uncover the intricate connection between movement and metabolic well-being, and discover how even small steps can pave the way towards a more vibrant and balanced life.

The Dynamics of Insulin Sensitivity and Physical Activity

Central to understanding the link between exercise and insulin sensitivity is comprehending the role of insulin itself. Insulin is a hormone produced by the pancreas, essential for regulating blood sugar levels. In individuals with diabetes, insulin sensitivity is diminished, leading to poor glucose control. This is where exercise emerges as a dynamic ally.

Engaging in regular physical activity enhances insulin sensitivity, facilitating the efficient transport of glucose from the bloodstream into cells. As muscles contract during exercise, they become more receptive to insulin's actions, allowing for improved glucose uptake. This process not only helps regulate blood sugar levels but also reduces the strain on the pancreas, potentially slowing the progression of diabetes.

The Transformative Power of Movement

Exercise goes beyond its impact on insulin sensitivity; it plays a pivotal role in shaping overall health. Let's explore some of the profound ways in which physical activity can positively influence our well-being:

Weight Management: One of the most visible effects of regular exercise is its ability to support weight management. Physical activity burns calories, contributing to a healthy energy balance. Additionally, as we engage in exercise, our bodies develop lean muscle mass, which in turn elevates our basal metabolic rate. This means that even when at rest, our bodies continue to burn calories more efficiently.

Cardiovascular Health: The heart is at the core of our circulatory system, and exercise is its ally in maintaining vitality. Regular physical activity strengthens the heart muscle, enhances circulation, and reduces the risk of cardiovascular diseases that often accompany diabetes.

Stress Reduction: Stress, a ubiquitous modern challenge, can significantly impact blood sugar levels. Engaging in physical activity triggers the release of endorphins, the body's natural mood enhancers, which help counteract stress and promote a sense of well-being.

Bone Health: Weight-bearing exercises, such as walking, jogging, and resistance training, stimulate bone growth and fortify bone density. This is particularly important for individuals with diabetes, who may be at a higher risk of bone-related issues.

Mind-Body Connection: Exercise nurtures the mind-body connection. Activities like yoga and tai chi combine movement with mindfulness, reducing stress and fostering emotional equilibrium.

The Journey of Incorporating Physical Activity

Embarking on a journey of regular exercise doesn't necessitate embarking on extreme training regimes. Rather, it involves incorporating movement into your daily routine in meaningful and sustainable ways:

Tailored Approach: Choose exercises that resonate with your preferences and physical condition. Whether it's brisk walking, cycling, swimming, or dancing, find activities that you enjoy.

Consistency Matters: Consistency is key. Aim for regularity in your exercise routine, gradually increasing the intensity and duration as your fitness improves.

Variety and Progression: Incorporate a variety of exercises to engage different muscle groups and prevent monotony. Additionally, challenge yourself with incremental increases in intensity to avoid plateaus.

Balancing Rest and Activity: While exercise is immensely beneficial, allowing your body time to recover is equally important. Balancing rest with activity prevents burnout and supports overall health.

Medical Guidance: For individuals with pre-existing medical conditions, consulting a healthcare professional before embarking on a new exercise regimen is advisable.

Lifestyle Integration: Infuse physical activity into your daily life. Opt for stairs instead of elevators, walk short distances instead of driving, and seize opportunities to move whenever possible.

In Conclusion: Empowerment through Movement

"Engage in regular exercise to improve insulin sensitivity and maintain a healthy weight" isn't just a recommendation; it's an invitation to embrace movement as a powerful tool in your wellness toolkit. By prioritising physical activity, you can unlock a cascade of benefits that extend beyond blood sugar regulation. With every step, you empower yourself to rewrite the narrative of your health, forging a path towards vitality, resilience, and a life imbued with well-being.

Chapter <3>

Mindful Carbohydrate Management: Navigating the Path to Balanced Energy

In the intricate dance of dietary choices, carbohydrates occupy a central role, influencing our energy levels, blood sugar regulation, and overall well-being. The chapter "Mindful Carbohydrate Management" guides us through the art of harnessing carbohydrates as a source of sustained energy while prioritizing blood sugar stability. As we journey through these insights, we'll uncover the nuances of carbohydrate selection, exploring the realm of complex carbs and the power of moderation.

The Carbohydrate Conundrum: Energy Source and Blood Sugar

Carbohydrates are the body's primary source of energy, providing the fuel necessary for various bodily functions. However, the type and quantity of carbohydrates consumed play a crucial role in determining how our bodies respond to glucose.

Simple carbohydrates, often found in refined sugars and processed foods, are rapidly digested and cause rapid spikes in blood sugar levels. This sudden surge triggers a subsequent crash in energy, leading to feelings of fatigue and cravings for more sugar. In individuals with diabetes, these fluctuations can be particularly challenging to manage.

On the other hand, complex carbohydrates, present in whole foods like grains, legumes, and vegetables, release energy gradually. This controlled release helps maintain steady blood sugar levels, providing sustained energy throughout the day. This chapter delves into the art of choosing complex carbohydrates to promote stable blood sugar and long-lasting vitality.

Complex Carbohydrates: Nourishing Sustenance

At the heart of mindful carbohydrate management lies the selection of complex carbohydrates. These carbohydrates are rich in dietary fiber, vitamins, and minerals, offering a range of health benefits beyond mere energy provision.

Whole Grains: Whole grains, such as brown rice, quinoa, and oats, are examples of complex carbohydrates. Unlike their refined counterparts, whole grains retain their bran and germ, which house essential nutrients and fibre. This fibre content not only slows down digestion but also supports gut health and contributes to a feeling of fullness, aiding in portion control.

Legumes: Beans, lentils, and chickpeas are nutritional powerhouses abundant in complex carbohydrates and protein. Their high fiber content aids digestion and helps modulate blood sugar levels. Legumes also boast a low glycemic index, meaning they have a gentle impact on blood sugar.

Vegetables: Non-starchy vegetables, including leafy greens, broccoli, and peppers, are excellent sources of complex carbohydrates. Their nutritional density, coupled with fiber content, makes them valuable allies in promoting stable blood sugar levels.

Mindful Consumption: The Art of Moderation

While complex carbohydrates provide a foundation of balanced energy, it's essential to approach their consumption mindfully. Portion control and awareness of total carbohydrate intake are integral aspects of effective carbohydrate management.

Glycemic Index: The glycemic index (GI) ranks carbohydrates based on how quickly they raise blood sugar levels. Foods with a low GI, such as most complex carbohydrates, have a gentler impact on blood sugar. Integrating foods with a low GI into your diet can aid in blood sugar regulation.

Balancing Act: The balance between carbohydrates, proteins, and fats in a meal influences how our bodies process glucose. Including a combination of these macronutrients can slow down the absorption of carbohydrates and help maintain stable blood sugar levels.

Monitoring and Learning: Regular monitoring of blood sugar levels can offer insights into how different foods impact your body. Over time, you'll become more attuned to your body's responses and can adjust your carbohydrate choices accordingly.

Mindful Eating: Slow down and savor your meals. Eating mindfully allows you to recognize feelings of fullness, preventing overconsumption.

Educated Choices: Understanding carbohydrate content in different foods empowers you to make informed decisions. Reading nutritional labels and seeking guidance from healthcare professionals can aid in this process.

In Conclusion: Crafting a Nourishing Carbohydrate Narrative

"Monitor carbohydrate intake and choose complex carbs that release energy gradually" encapsulates a philosophy of embracing carbohydrates as allies in our pursuit of vitality. By thoughtfully selecting complex carbohydrates and managing portion sizes, you can navigate the intricate realm of blood sugar regulation while nurturing sustained energy levels. As you embark on this journey of mindful carbohydrate management, remember that each choice you make contributes to the intricate tapestry of your well-being. Through balance and awareness, you can create a narrative of health that is rich, vibrant, and harmonious.

Chapter <4>

Hydration Habits: Quenching the Path to Wellness through Adequate Hydration

In the symphony of well-being, hydration stands as a fundamental note, shaping the harmony of our bodily functions. The chapter "Hydration Habits" takes us on a journey through the vital role that staying hydrated plays in supporting kidney function and contributing to effective blood sugar control. As we delve into the nuances of hydration, we'll uncover the intricate dance between fluids, kidneys, and glucose regulation, illuminating the path to a more balanced and vibrant life.

Fluids and Kidney Function: Nurturing Vital Filtration

The kidneys, two remarkable bean-shaped organs, serve as the body's natural filtration system. They play a pivotal role in removing waste products, balancing electrolytes, and maintaining fluid equilibrium. Adequate hydration is paramount for the optimal functioning of these vital organs.

When we are well-hydrated, the kidneys are better equipped to efficiently filter waste and toxins from the bloodstream. This not only supports overall health but also ensures that other bodily systems can operate at their best. As we explore hydration habits, it becomes clear that water is not merely a beverage; it's an elixir that nurtures the body's intricate machinery.

Hydration and Blood Sugar Control: Balancing Glucose Levels

Beyond kidney function, staying hydrated also influences blood sugar control, a particularly relevant aspect for individuals with diabetes. The relationship between hydration and glucose regulation is multifaceted, involving both hydration's impact on insulin sensitivity and its role in diluting excess glucose.

Insulin Sensitivity: Hydration plays a role in enhancing insulin sensitivity, making cells more responsive to the hormone's actions. Improved insulin sensitivity can lead to more effective glucose uptake by cells, helping to maintain stable blood sugar levels.

Dilution Effect: Hydration contributes to the dilution of excess glucose in the bloodstream. Drinking water helps flush out glucose through urine, reducing the risk of hyperglycemia (high blood sugar).

Practical Hydration Practices

Adopting effective hydration practices involves more than simply drinking water; it's about cultivating a lifestyle that nurtures your body's fluid needs. Here are some practical tips to weave hydration into your daily routine:

Water as a Constant Companion: Carry a reusable water bottle with you to encourage regular sips throughout the day. This practice helps prevent dehydration and supports consistent kidney function.

Hydration Signals: Listen to your body's signals of thirst. Thirst is a natural indicator that your body requires fluids. Respond to these signals promptly to maintain optimal hydration levels.

Strategic Hydration: Spread your water intake throughout the day rather than consuming large amounts at once. This approach helps maintain steady hydration levels.

Hydrating Foods: Incorporate water-rich foods into your diet, such as fruits (watermelon, cucumbers) and vegetables (lettuce, celery). These foods contribute to your overall fluid intake.

Monitoring Urine Color: Monitoring the color of your urine can provide insights into your hydration status. Pale yellow urine indicates good hydration, while dark yellow or amber suggests the need for more fluids.

Caffeine and Alcohol Consideration: Be mindful of the diuretic effects of caffeine and alcohol, which can increase fluid loss. Compensate by drinking additional water if you consume these beverages.

Hydration and Diabetes Management

For individuals with diabetes, effective hydration is a valuable tool in blood sugar control. Here's how to align hydration with diabetes management:

Consultation with Healthcare Professionals: Seek guidance from healthcare professionals to determine your individual hydration needs, considering factors such as diabetes medication and overall health status.

Integration with Meal Plans: Incorporate hydration as a cornerstone of your meal plans. Drink water before, during, and after meals to support digestion and blood sugar regulation.

Hydration during Exercise: Stay well-hydrated during physical activity, as exercise can increase fluid loss. This is especially important for individuals with diabetes, as maintaining hydration aids in stable blood sugar levels.

In Conclusion: Nurturing Wellness Drop by Drop

"Stay hydrated to support kidney function and aid in blood sugar control" encapsulates the profound significance of fluid intake in nurturing holistic health. By understanding the relationship between hydration, kidney function, and blood sugar regulation, you can embark on a journey of self-care that ripples through every aspect of your well-being. As you incorporate mindful hydration practices into your daily routine, remember that each sip is a step towards optimal vitality—an investment in a life that is well-nourished, balanced, and flourishing.

Chapter <5>

Strategic Meal Timing: Crafting Blood Sugar Harmony Through Thoughtful Eating

In the intricate orchestration of our health, the timing of meals emerges as a conductor, shaping the rhythm of our energy levels and blood sugar stability. The chapter "Strategic Meal Timing" guides us through the art of synchronising meal patterns to prevent abrupt spikes and crashes in blood sugar levels. As we journey through this exploration, we'll uncover the delicate balance between meal frequency, portion control, and blood sugar regulation, uncovering a path towards sustained vitality and equilibrium.

The Dance of Blood Sugar: Understanding Spikes and Crashes

Blood sugar levels, known as glucose, play a pivotal role in maintaining the body's energy reserves. However, the body's response to meals, especially those high in carbohydrates, can lead to rapid surges and subsequent crashes in blood sugar. These fluctuations can be particularly challenging for individuals with diabetes, who aim to achieve stable and controlled glucose levels.

Meal Timing's Influence: Strategic meal timing offers a method to manage these fluctuations. By distributing your food intake throughout the day, you can modulate the release of glucose into the bloodstream, preventing sharp spikes and crashes.

The Power of Frequent, Smaller Meals

One of the key principles of strategic meal timing involves opting for smaller, frequent meals instead of a traditional three-meals-a-day pattern. This approach has several advantages when it comes to blood sugar regulation and overall well-being:

Balanced Energy: Consuming smaller, frequent meals helps maintain a steady supply of energy throughout the day. This approach prevents the energy slumps that often accompany larger, infrequent meals.

Improved Insulin Response: Eating smaller portions at regular intervals allows the body to manage glucose more efficiently. The pancreas can release insulin in a controlled manner, preventing sudden spikes in blood sugar levels.

Portion Control: Smaller meals naturally encourage portion control, reducing the likelihood of overeating and excess glucose intake.

Digestive Ease: Frequent, smaller meals can ease the digestive process, allowing the body to absorb nutrients more effectively and preventing digestive discomfort.

The Balance Between Nutrients

Strategic meal timing goes hand in hand with the composition of your meals. To harness its benefits effectively, it's essential to consider not only the frequency of meals but also the balance between macronutrients—carbohydrates, proteins, and fats.

Carbohydrate Distribution: Distribute your carbohydrate intake evenly across your smaller meals. This approach prevents a concentrated surge of glucose entering the bloodstream, supporting steady blood sugar levels.

Protein-Powered Satiety: Including lean proteins in each meal provides satiety, reducing the risk of overeating and promoting stable energy levels.

Healthy Fats: Incorporate healthy fats, such as those found in nuts, seeds, and avocados, to slow down the absorption of nutrients and prevent rapid glucose spikes.

Practical Meal Timing Strategies

Implementing strategic meal timing requires a thoughtful and adaptable approach. Here are some practical strategies to consider:

Personalised Schedule: Tailor your meal frequency to your personal schedule and preferences. While some individuals thrive on three main meals and a snack, others might prefer a series of smaller, more frequent meals.

Mindful Planning: Plan your meals in advance, ensuring that each one contains a balance of nutrients. This practice prevents impulsive choices that can lead to unbalanced glucose levels.

Snack Selection: Choose nutrient-dense snacks that align with your blood sugar goals. Opt for whole fruits, Greek yoghourt, or a handful of nuts as wholesome options.

Hydration Habits: Integrate adequate hydration between meals to support digestion and overall well-being.

Blood Sugar Monitoring: Regularly monitor your blood sugar levels to observe how different meal timing strategies affect your glucose responses. This knowledge empowers you to fine-tune your approach.

The Synergy of Timing and Wellness

"Opt for smaller, frequent meals to prevent spikes and crashes in blood sugar levels" encapsulates the essence of strategic meal timing as a tool to shape your well-being. By distributing your food intake strategically and aligning it with nutrient balance, you can cultivate a harmonious relationship with your blood sugar levels. As you embrace the dance of meal timing, remember that each choice you make contributes to the symphony of your health—a symphony that resonates with vitality, equilibrium, and a life that is nourished in every sense.

Chapter <6>

Sugar Scrutiny: Unveiling the Hidden Sweetness for Informed Dietary Choices

In the realm of nutritional exploration, few topics are as pivotal as our relationship with sugar. The chapter "Sugar Scrutiny" invites us to embark on a journey of meticulous label reading and conscious decision-making, as we uncover the hidden sugars that infiltrate our diets and learn to reduce added sugars to curb excessive glucose intake. Through this exploration, we illuminate the intricate connection between sugar consumption, blood sugar levels, and overall wellness.

The Sugar Landscape: From Pleasure to Caution

Sugar, a source of pleasure and energy, is omnipresent in our modern diets. Yet, the ease with which it can be consumed often obscures the potential risks it poses, particularly for individuals concerned with blood sugar control and diabetes management. Sugar can lead to rapid spikes in blood glucose levels, placing stress on the body's ability to regulate these levels effectively.

Understanding the nuances of sugar consumption involves differentiating between natural sugars present in whole foods (such as fruits) and added sugars found in processed and packaged products. The focus of "Sugar Scrutiny" lies on added sugars, which often hide behind an array of names on labels. By cultivating a discerning eye for labels and reducing our consumption of added sugars, we can navigate the complex sugar landscape with greater awareness.

Label Reading: The Art of Unmasking Hidden Sugars

Reading labels meticulously is a skill that empowers us to make informed dietary choices. Added sugars can manifest under various guises, from sucrose and high fructose corn syrup to more covert names like dextrose and maltodextrin. Recognizing these aliases is the first step towards unveiling the true sugar content of packaged products.

Ingredients List: Delve into the ingredients list to identify added sugars. Look for terms like "syrup," "nectar," and anything ending in "-ose," as they often indicate added sugars.

Nutrition Facts: Pay attention to the "Total Sugars" listed in the nutrition facts panel. This figure encompasses both natural and added sugars. To differentiate, refer to the "Added Sugars" subsection, which reveals the amount of sugars that aren't naturally occurring in the food.

Serving Size Awareness: Keep serving sizes in mind while interpreting sugar content. Sometimes, a product might seem low in sugar, but the serving size could be smaller than what you actually consume.

Sugar Content per 100g: For easier comparison, consider the sugar content per 100 grams. This standardisation helps you gauge the sugar content across different products.

Reducing Added Sugars: A Journey of Empowerment

The journey towards reducing added sugars is an exercise in empowerment. By making conscious choices, you regain control over your sugar intake and contribute to more balanced blood sugar levels. Here are practical steps to help you embark on this journey:

Whole Foods Embrace: Prioritise whole foods over processed ones. Whole fruits, vegetables, lean proteins, and whole grains provide essential nutrients without the added sugars found in many packaged products.

Cooking Mastery: Preparing meals at home allows you to control the ingredients, ensuring that added sugars are kept to a minimum.

Sugar-Free Alternatives: Explore natural sugar substitutes like stevia, erythritol, and monk fruit. However, use these substitutes in moderation and consult healthcare professionals if you have any concerns.

Label Comparisons: When choosing packaged products, compare labels to identify those with lower added sugar content. Opt for products that provide essential nutrients without unnecessary sweeteners.

Mindful Indulgence: If you choose to indulge in sweet treats, do so mindfully and in moderation. Consider sharing desserts or opting for smaller portions.

Education and Advocacy

"Sugar Scrutiny" extends beyond personal choices; it also advocates for greater transparency and education regarding sugar content in food products. By raising awareness and demanding clearer labelling practices, we can collectively create an environment where individuals can make more informed choices about their dietary intake.

In Conclusion: Empowerment through Conscious Choices

"Read labels meticulously and reduce added sugars in your diet to curb excessive glucose intake" encapsulates a journey of empowerment, where every label read and sugar-conscious choice brings you closer to balanced blood sugar levels and overall well-being. By unmasking hidden sugars and nurturing a discerning relationship with sweeteners, you shape a narrative of health that's guided by informed decisions. Remember that each step taken in the realm of sugar scrutiny is a step towards vitality—a stride towards a life that's both sweet and savoured, yet thoughtfully balanced.

Chapter <7>

Portion Control: A Balanced Culinary Symphony for Steady Blood Sugar Levels

In the culinary ballet of health, portion control emerges as the choreographer, guiding the graceful steps towards maintaining steady blood sugar levels and preventing overindulgence. The chapter "Portion Control" invites us to master the art of mindful eating, as we navigate the delicate balance between satisfaction and restraint. Through this exploration, we'll uncover the profound impact of portion sizes on blood sugar regulation and discover strategies to foster a harmonious relationship with food.

The Dynamics of Portions and Blood Sugar Levels

Portion control isn't merely a weight management strategy; it's a potent tool for stabilising blood sugar levels. The quantity of food we consume in a single sitting influences the body's response, particularly for individuals concerned with blood sugar management. Oversized portions can lead to a surge in blood glucose, placing strain on the body's ability to process and regulate these levels effectively.

By embracing portion control, we strike a chord of moderation that resonates through our metabolic processes. The goal is to enjoy meals that satisfy both hunger and nutritional needs without triggering rapid fluctuations in blood sugar.

Mindful Eating: The Essence of Portion Control

Mindful eating forms the cornerstone of effective portion control. It's a practice that involves engaging all your senses, savouring each bite, and attuning to your body's hunger and satiety cues. Here's how mindful eating intertwines with portion control:

Sensory Engagement: Before you take the first bite, engage your senses. Observe the colours, textures, and aromas of your food. This awareness enhances the dining experience and encourages a slower, more conscious pace of eating.

Savour Each Bite: Take your time to chew and appreciate the flavours of your food. Eating slowly allows your brain to receive signals of fullness, preventing overeating.

Hunger Signals: Tune in to your body's hunger signals. Eat when you're genuinely hungry and stop when you feel comfortably satisfied, not stuffed.

Distraction-Free Dining: Minimise distractions while eating. Turn off screens and focus solely on the meal in front of you. This practice encourages mindful enjoyment and prevents mindless overconsumption.

Strategies for Portion Control

Effective portion control doesn't involve deprivation; it's about relishing food while being attuned to your body's signals. Here are strategies to help you master the art of portion control:

Plate Composition: Visualise your plate as a canvas. Aim to fill half your plate with non-starchy vegetables, a quarter with lean protein, and the remaining quarter with complex carbohydrates.

Use Smaller Plates: Opt for smaller plates and bowls. When you serve food on a smaller surface, it appears more substantial, promoting satisfaction with smaller portions.

Pre-Portioned Snacks: When snacking, portion out snacks into small containers or bags. This prevents mindless munching and helps you keep track of portion sizes.

Mindful Servings: Serve yourself a smaller portion initially, and if you're still hungry after finishing, wait a few minutes before deciding if you need more. This practice allows your brain to catch up with your stomach's cues.

Beverage Awareness: Be mindful of beverage portions, particularly when consuming sugary drinks. Opt for smaller glasses and consider diluting juices or choosing water to hydrate.

Listening to Your Body: The Core Principle

Amidst the tactics and strategies, the core principle of portion control remains listening to your body. Your body communicates its needs through hunger and fullness cues. Trusting these cues and honouring your body's signals is the essence of portion control.

Blood Sugar Regulation and Beyond

"Be mindful of portion sizes to avoid overeating and maintain steady blood sugar levels" encapsulates a journey of balance that transcends blood sugar regulation. By aligning portion sizes with your body's needs, you foster a relationship with food that nourishes both body and soul. Through mindful eating, you cultivate a symphony of well-being that resonates with vitality, mindfulness, and a life that's harmoniously nourished.

Chapter <8>

Fibre Incorporation: Weaving Nutritional Resilience with High-Fibre Choices

In the intricate tapestry of nutrition, fibre emerges as a thread of remarkable significance. The chapter "Fiber Incorporation" invites us to explore the multifaceted benefits of including high-fibre foods in our diets. By regulating digestion, slowing glucose absorption, and promoting satiety, fibre becomes a cornerstone of balanced well-being. As we delve into this exploration, we'll uncover the profound impact of fibre on blood sugar regulation and overall vitality.

The Fibre Spectrum: From Soluble to Insoluble

Fibre, found exclusively in plant-based foods, can be categorised into two types: soluble and insoluble. Both types offer distinct advantages when it comes to supporting blood sugar regulation, digestion, and overall health.

Soluble Fibre: This type of fibre dissolves in water to form a gel-like substance in the digestive tract. Soluble fibre helps regulate blood sugar levels by slowing down the absorption of glucose. It also contributes to a feeling of fullness, which can aid in portion control.

Insoluble Fibre: Insoluble fibre adds bulk to stool, aiding in regular bowel movements and preventing constipation. While it doesn't directly impact blood sugar, its contribution to digestive health indirectly supports overall well-being.

Blood Sugar Regulation: The Fibre Connection

The impact of fibre on blood sugar regulation is one of its most notable attributes. By influencing the pace at which glucose is absorbed, fibre offers a natural mechanism to manage blood sugar levels.

Glucose Absorption Delays: Soluble fibre's gel-like nature slows down the absorption of glucose in the digestive tract. This measured absorption prevents rapid spikes in blood sugar, promoting more stable levels over time.

Balancing Meal Composition: Including high-fibre foods in meals can temper the overall glycemic response. The presence of fibre mitigates the impact of carbohydrates on blood sugar, promoting a smoother glucose curve.

Sustained Energy: The gradual release of glucose facilitated by fibre-rich foods leads to sustained energy levels. This effect is particularly valuable for individuals striving to maintain consistent energy throughout the day.

Promoting Satiety: A Natural Appetite Regulator

Fiber's role in promoting satiety—feeling full and satisfied after a meal—can be a game-changer for portion control and overall dietary balance.

Appetite Suppression: High-fibre foods require more chewing and take longer to digest. This process sends signals to the brain that you're full, helping prevent overeating.

Portion Control: By promoting a feeling of fullness, fibre encourages portion control. Smaller portions can lead to controlled calorie intake and more stable blood sugar levels.

Digestive Resilience: Nurturing Gut Health

Beyond its role in blood sugar regulation, fibre supports digestive health in various ways:

Bowel Regularity: Insoluble fibre adds bulk to stool, preventing constipation and promoting regular bowel movements.

Microbiome Support: Fibre serves as a prebiotic, providing nourishment for beneficial gut bacteria. A thriving gut microbiome is linked to improved digestion and overall health.

Practical Fiber Incorporation Strategies

Incorporating high-fibre foods into your diet doesn't require drastic changes; it involves thoughtful choices and an awareness of fibre-rich options:

Whole Grains: Opt for whole grains like quinoa, brown rice, and whole wheat bread instead of refined grains. These grains retain their fibre content, providing more sustained energy.

Legumes: Beans, lentils, and chickpeas are rich sources of soluble and insoluble fibre. They can be integrated into soups, stews, salads, and various dishes.

Fruits and Vegetables: Non-starchy vegetables like broccoli, spinach, and Brussels sprouts are excellent sources of fibre. Whole fruits, especially those with edible skins, also contribute to your fibre intake.

Seeds and Nuts: Chia seeds, flaxseeds, almonds, and walnuts are packed with fibre and healthy fats. They can be added to smoothies, oatmeal, or yoghurt.

Gradual Incorporation: Introduce fibre-rich foods gradually to allow your digestive system to adjust. Rapidly increasing fibre intake can initially cause discomfort.

Hydration: Fibre works optimally when accompanied by adequate hydration. Drinking water throughout the day supports the movement of fibre through the digestive tract.

In Conclusion: Nourishing with Nature's Bounty

"Include high-fibre foods to regulate digestion, slow glucose absorption, and promote satiety" encapsulates the essence of harnessing nature's bounty for balanced well-being. By embracing fibre-rich choices, you create a narrative of vitality that resonates with sustained energy, mindful satisfaction, and resilience in blood sugar control. Remember that each fibre-rich choice you make is a step towards cultivating a life imbued with nourishment—a life woven with the threads of health, balance, and vibrant harmony.

Chapter <9>

Healthy Fats Selection: Elevating Wellness Through Thoughtful Fat Choices

In the realm of nutrition, the spotlight often falls on fats—a macronutrient of intrigue and diversity. The chapter "Healthy Fats Selection" extends an invitation to explore the nuances of fat choices, guiding us towards the embrace of unsaturated fats over saturated ones. By making mindful choices in fat consumption, we not only support cardiovascular health but also enhance insulin sensitivity—a harmony of well-being that resonates deeply. As we journey through this exploration, we'll unveil the intricate interplay between fats, health, and balance, shaping a narrative of vitality and resilience.

Fat Diversity: A Spectrum of Impact

Fats are more than mere calorie sources; they're influential players in the intricate orchestra of health. The categories of fats—saturated, unsaturated, and trans fats—possess distinct effects on the body, with unsaturated fats standing as champions of cardiovascular wellness and metabolic balance.

Saturated Fats: These fats, often found in animal products and some tropical oils, have been linked to higher levels of LDL (low-density lipoprotein) cholesterol—the "bad" cholesterol associated with cardiovascular risk. Excessive consumption of saturated fats can potentially impair insulin sensitivity, a concern for individuals with diabetes.

Unsaturated Fats: Unsaturated fats, in contrast, offer a contrasting narrative of health. Found in plant-based sources and fatty fish, these fats include monounsaturated and polyunsaturated fats. They contribute to the elevation of HDL (high-density lipoprotein) cholesterol—the "good" cholesterol that supports cardiovascular well-being. Unsaturated fats have also been associated with improved insulin sensitivity, a crucial factor in blood sugar regulation.

The Cardiovascular Connection: Elevating Heart Health

Healthy fat selection is intimately connected with cardiovascular well-being. By favouring unsaturated fats, we contribute to the preservation of heart health and reduce the risk of cardiovascular diseases. Here's how the journey towards healthier fats supports the heart:

Cholesterol Regulation: Unsaturated fats have the power to lower LDL cholesterol levels, helping to maintain a balanced cholesterol profile.

Inflammation Mitigation: Chronic inflammation is a contributing factor to cardiovascular diseases. Unsaturated fats possess anti-inflammatory properties, working to mitigate this risk.

Endothelial Function: The inner lining of blood vessels, called the endothelium, plays a crucial role in cardiovascular health. Unsaturated fats support the healthy function of the endothelium, promoting better blood flow.

Insulin Sensitivity Enhancement: The Metabolic Advantage

For individuals navigating diabetes, the role of fat selection extends to insulin sensitivity—a cornerstone of blood sugar regulation. Insulin sensitivity determines how effectively cells respond to insulin, facilitating the entry of glucose into cells for energy use.

Unsaturated fats, particularly omega-3 fatty acids found in fatty fish like salmon, have been associated with improved insulin sensitivity. These fats support better glucose uptake by cells, contributing to more stable blood sugar levels.

Strategies for Healthy Fat Selection

Incorporating healthy fats into your diet involves making conscious choices that align with your well-being goals. Here are practical strategies for navigating fat choices:

Cooking Oils: Opt for oils high in unsaturated fats for cooking and dressings. Olive oil, avocado oil, and canola oil are excellent choices.

Fatty Fish: Integrate fatty fish like salmon, mackerel, and sardines into your diet. These fish are rich in omega-3 fatty acids, which offer cardiovascular and insulin sensitivity benefits.

Nuts and Seeds: Almonds, walnuts, chia seeds, and flaxseeds are sources of healthy fats. They can be added to meals, snacks, or smoothies.

Avocado: This creamy fruit is abundant in monounsaturated fats and offers versatile culinary possibilities, from spreads to salads.

Lean Proteins: Choose lean protein sources, such as poultry and legumes, and pair them with unsaturated fats for a balanced meal.

Reading Labels: When selecting packaged foods, read labels to identify the types of fats used. Opt for products with healthier fat profiles.

A Holistic Culmination: Heart Health and Metabolic Balance

"Choose unsaturated fats over saturated ones to support cardiovascular health and insulin sensitivity" encapsulates a journey that intertwines heart health and metabolic equilibrium. By embracing unsaturated fats, you craft a narrative of resilience—one that resonates with the vibrant symphony of a heart in harmony and glucose regulation at its best. Remember that each

thoughtful fat choice is a note in the composition of your health—a note
that reverberates with vitality, awareness, and a life that is nourished on
multiple levels.

Chapter <10>

Healthy Fats Selection: Nurturing Wellness Through Mindful Fat Choices

In the symphony of nutrition, fats compose a crucial melody that resonates
throughout our health. The chapter "Healthy Fats Selection" beckons us to
explore the art of fat selection, urging us to opt for unsaturated fats over
saturated ones. This mindful choice not only nurtures cardiovascular health
but also fosters improved insulin sensitivity—a harmonious rhythm of
well-being. As we delve into this exploration, we'll illuminate the intricate
dance between fats, health, and balance, crafting a narrative that exudes
vitality and resilience.

The Spectrum of Fats: Shaping Our Health

Fats are more than just energy providers; they play a pivotal role in our
physiological harmony. Fats come in various forms—saturated,
unsaturated, and trans fats—each contributing distinct notes to our health.
Among them, unsaturated fats emerge as champions of cardiovascular
well-being and metabolic balance.

Saturated Fats: Often found in animal products and certain oils,
saturated fats have been linked to elevated levels of LDL (low-density

lipoprotein) cholesterol—the "bad" cholesterol known to increase cardiovascular risk. Excessive intake of saturated fats can potentially hinder insulin sensitivity, a concern for those managing diabetes.

Unsaturated Fats: On the other hand, unsaturated fats present a symphony of health. Found in plant-based sources and fatty fish, these fats include both monounsaturated and polyunsaturated fats. They contribute to the elevation of HDL (high-density lipoprotein) cholesterol—the "good" cholesterol that supports heart well-being. Unsaturated fats have also been associated with heightened insulin sensitivity, a crucial factor in blood sugar management.

A Tune of Cardiovascular Health: Elevating Heart Well-Being

The choices we make regarding fats are deeply intertwined with our cardiovascular health. Embracing unsaturated fats leads to the preservation of heart wellness and a reduction in the risk of cardiovascular ailments. Here's how this virtuous journey unfolds:

Cholesterol Regulation: Unsaturated fats possess the remarkable ability to lower LDL cholesterol levels, contributing to a balanced cholesterol profile that supports heart health.

Inflammation Management: Chronic inflammation is a significant contributor to cardiovascular diseases. Unsaturated fats exhibit anti-inflammatory properties that assist in managing this risk.

Endothelial Harmony: The endothelium, the inner lining of blood vessels, plays a pivotal role in heart health. Unsaturated fats help maintain the endothelium's function, promoting improved blood flow and overall cardiovascular resilience.

Elevating Insulin Sensitivity: A Metabolic Marvel

For individuals navigating the terrain of diabetes, the implications of fat selection extend to insulin sensitivity—a critical component of blood sugar regulation. Insulin sensitivity dictates how effectively cells respond to insulin, facilitating the entrance of glucose into cells for energy utilisation.

**Unsaturated fats, particularly omega-3 fatty acids found in fatty fish like salmon, have been linked to enhanced insulin sensitivity. These fats bolster the body's ability to uptake glucose, ultimately leading to more stable blood sugar levels.

Strategies for Embracing Healthy Fats

Incorporating healthy fats into our diets necessitates conscious choices that align with our well-being aspirations. Here are pragmatic strategies for navigating the landscape of fat selection:

Culinary Oils: Opt for oils rich in unsaturated fats for cooking and dressing. Olive oil, avocado oil, and canola oil are splendid choices that infuse dishes with health-enhancing properties.

Fatty Fish: Integrate fatty fish such as salmon, mackerel, and sardines into your diet. These fish are brimming with omega-3 fatty acids that offer both cardiovascular benefits and improved insulin sensitivity.

Nutty Delights: Almonds, walnuts, chia seeds, and flaxseeds are treasure troves of healthy fats. Sprinkle these nutritional gems onto meals, snacks, or into smoothies for a delightful crunch and wellness boost.

The Avocado Affair: Avocado, with its creamy allure, is rich in monounsaturated fats. It presents an array of culinary possibilities, from spreads to salads, all contributing to heart health.

Lean Proteins: When choosing proteins, lean options such as poultry and legumes offer a balanced foundation for a meal. Pairing them with unsaturated fats creates a harmony of nourishment.

Label Literacy: When perusing packaged goods, inspect labels to discern the types of fats used. Prioritise products featuring healthier fat profiles.

A Harmonious Culmination: Heart and Metabolic Flourish

"Choose unsaturated fats over saturated ones to support cardiovascular health and insulin sensitivity" encapsulates a journey that intertwines heart vitality and metabolic resilience. By embracing unsaturated fats, you script a narrative of strength—one that echoes with the melodious cadence of a heart in tune and glucose management at its finest. Remember that every intentional choice towards healthier fats composes a note in the symphony of your well-being—a note that reverberates with vitality, mindfulness, and a life that is nourished on multiple levels.

Chapter <11>

Stress Management: Cultivating Calm Amidst the Storm for Balanced Blood Sugar Levels

In the intricate tapestry of health, stress emerges as a potent thread that can weave both chaos and harmony. The chapter "Stress Management" extends an invitation to explore the art of finding reprieve within relaxation techniques, such as meditation and deep breathing. By harnessing these tools, we embark on a journey to quell stress-induced blood sugar spikes, fostering a realm of balance that resonates deeply. As we delve into this exploration, we'll illuminate the intricate dance between stress, blood sugar regulation, and tranquillity—a dance that shapes a narrative of vitality and serenity.

Stress's Impact on Blood Sugar: The Unseen Culprit

The interplay between stress and blood sugar is a complex symphony. Stress, whether triggered by emotional upheavals, work pressure, or life's demands, has the potential to send blood sugar levels on a roller-coaster ride. The body's "fight or flight" response to stress often involves the release of hormones like cortisol and adrenaline. These hormones can lead to a surge in blood sugar levels, priming the body for action.

For individuals with diabetes or those aiming for stable blood sugar levels, stress-induced spikes can pose a significant challenge. The delicate dance between hormones and glucose requires careful navigation—one that relaxation techniques can masterfully guide.

The Tranquil Refuge: Meditation and Deep Breathing

In the realm of stress management, meditation and deep breathing stand as beacons of tranquillity. These practices provide a sanctuary amidst life's hustle, offering a pathway to calm the mind, soothe the body, and regulate blood sugar levels.

Meditation: Meditation, whether guided or mindfulness-based, involves focusing the mind on the present moment. This practice cultivates awareness, reduces stress, and contributes to a state of mental equilibrium. Research indicates that regular meditation can improve insulin sensitivity and regulate blood sugar levels.

Deep Breathing: Deep breathing exercises harness the power of the breath to induce relaxation. Slow, deliberate inhalations and exhalations signal the body to activate the parasympathetic nervous system—a state of "rest and digest." This shift counteracts the stress-induced "fight or flight" response and promotes blood sugar stability.

The Physiology of Relaxation: Navigating Stress's Impact

The physiological mechanisms through which meditation and deep breathing influence blood sugar levels are profound:

Cortisol Regulation: Meditation and deep breathing have been linked to cortisol reduction—the hormone responsible for stress-related blood sugar spikes. By moderating cortisol levels, these practices help maintain stable glucose levels.

Insulin Sensitivity Enhancement: Regular relaxation techniques are associated with improved insulin sensitivity. This enhancement enables cells to more effectively absorb glucose, preventing excessive glucose in the bloodstream.

Nervous System Balance: Meditation and deep breathing activate the parasympathetic nervous system—a state of relaxation that counters the stress-induced dominance of the sympathetic nervous system. This balance supports blood sugar regulation.

Strategies for Stress-Relief Integration

Integrating relaxation techniques into your routine requires intention and commitment. Here are strategies to weave these practices into your daily life:

Mindful Moments: Dedicate short moments throughout the day to mindfulness. Engage in a few minutes of deep breathing or meditation to reset your stress response.

Designated Time: Set aside a specific time for relaxation practices. This can be in the morning, during breaks, or before bedtime—whichever aligns with your schedule.

Guided Resources: Utilise guided meditation apps or online resources to ease into meditation. These resources provide structure and guidance, making the practice more accessible.

Progressive Relaxation: Incorporate progressive muscle relaxation into your routine. This involves tensing and then releasing each muscle group, promoting overall relaxation.

Breathing Exercises: Explore deep breathing techniques such as diaphragmatic breathing or box breathing. These exercises can be done anywhere and have an immediate calming effect.

Reflective Practices: Combine relaxation with journaling or gratitude exercises. This combination enhances the emotional benefits of stress relief.

Cultivating a Serene Symphony: Stress, Harmony, and Blood Sugar

"Employ relaxation techniques like meditation and deep breathing to lower stress-induced blood sugar spikes" encapsulates a journey of weaving calm into the fabric of daily life. By embracing meditation and deep breathing, you craft a narrative of resilience—one that resonates with harmony amidst the storm of stress and blood sugar management. Each mindful breath and tranquil moment you invest is a note in the symphony of your well-being—a note that reverberates with vitality, peace, and a life that is nourished by serenity.

Chapter <12>

Adequate Sleep Routine: Nurturing Wellness Through Restful Slumber

In the intricate composition of health, sleep takes centre stage as a crucial melody that orchestrates well-being. The chapter "Adequate Sleep Routine" invites us to explore the art of prioritising sufficient sleep—a practice that transcends rest to weave vitality into our metabolic, hormonal, and overall equilibrium. As we delve into this exploration, we'll illuminate the profound interplay between sleep, metabolism, and well-being, crafting a narrative of rejuvenation and holistic health.

The Sleep Connection: Unveiling a Crucial Tapestry

Sleep is far more than a nightly respite; it's a foundational pillar upon which our health and vitality are built. The intricate dance between sleep and health encompasses a symphony of physiological processes that extend far beyond mere rest.

Metabolism Harmony: Sleep plays a pivotal role in metabolism—a complex web of processes that govern energy utilisation. Insufficient sleep disrupts metabolic balance, potentially leading to weight gain and insulin resistance.

Hormonal Synchrony: Sleep governs hormonal harmony, influencing the secretion of hormones like cortisol, insulin, and growth hormone. Adequate sleep contributes to a balanced hormonal profile that supports overall health.

Cognitive Restoration: Sleep is a time of cognitive rejuvenation. During sleep, the brain processes the day's events, enhances memory, and prepares for the challenges ahead.

The Sleep-Insulin Connection: Regulating Blood Sugar

The relationship between sleep and blood sugar regulation is profound, particularly for individuals managing diabetes or aiming for stable blood sugar levels.

Insulin Sensitivity: Sufficient sleep enhances insulin sensitivity—the body's responsiveness to insulin. Improved insulin sensitivity aids in the effective uptake of glucose by cells, maintaining stable blood sugar levels.

Hormonal Balance: Sleep influences the release of hormones that impact blood sugar, including insulin and cortisol. Disrupted sleep can lead to imbalanced hormone levels, contributing to blood sugar fluctuations.

Metabolic Momentum: Adequate sleep supports a well-functioning metabolism. Sleep deprivation disrupts this harmony, potentially leading to irregular glucose metabolism.

Strategies for Cultivating a Sleep Oasis

Cultivating an adequate sleep routine requires intention and the incorporation of healthy sleep practices. Here are strategies to foster restful slumber:

Consistent Sleep Schedule: Establish a regular sleep schedule, aiming for the same bedtime and wake-up time every day—even on weekends.

Sleep Environment: Create a sleep-conducive environment that's comfortable, dark, and quiet. Invest in a comfortable mattress and pillows to enhance sleep quality.

Digital Detox: Minimise screen exposure before bedtime. The blue light emitted by screens can disrupt the production of melatonin—a sleep-inducing hormone.

Relaxation Rituals: Engage in calming activities before bed, such as reading, meditation, or gentle stretching. These practices signal your body that it's time to wind down.

Limit Stimulants: Avoid caffeine and heavy meals close to bedtime. These can interfere with sleep quality and disrupt your sleep routine.

Physical Activity: Engage in regular physical activity, but avoid intense exercise close to bedtime. Regular exercise supports better sleep quality.

Balancing Naps: While short daytime naps can offer rejuvenation, avoid extended naps that could disrupt nighttime sleep.

Technology Management: Utilise sleep-tracking apps or wearable devices to monitor sleep patterns and identify areas for improvement.

Nurturing Sleep's Role in Well-Being: A Holistic Approach

"Prioritise sufficient sleep to aid metabolism, hormonal balance, and overall well-being" encapsulates a journey of embracing sleep as a cornerstone of holistic health. By valuing and fostering restful slumber, you weave a narrative of resilience—one that harmonises metabolism, hormones, and vitality. Each night of rejuvenating sleep and each conscious sleep-enhancing choice you make is a note in the symphony of your well-being—a note that resonates with vitality, balance, and a life that is truly well-rested.

Chapter <13>

Regular Monitoring: Illuminating Blood Sugar Pathways for Informed Lifestyle Mastery

In the intricate labyrinth of health, monitoring stands as a beacon of illumination—a compass that guides us through the dynamic terrain of blood sugar regulation. The chapter "Regular Monitoring" extends an invitation to explore the art of keeping track of blood sugar levels—a practice that transcends numbers to shape a narrative of empowerment and informed decision-making. As we delve into this exploration, we'll unveil the profound impact of regular monitoring on blood sugar mastery, revealing patterns that become stepping stones to tailored lifestyle adjustments.

The Monitoring Paradigm: Beyond Numbers and Into Understanding

Monitoring blood sugar levels is not just about numbers on a metre; it's a journey that unfolds layers of insight into your body's unique responses. By keeping a watchful eye on these levels, you unveil patterns that whisper stories of how various factors—food choices, physical activity, stress, and more—contribute to your blood sugar symphony.

Personalised Insight: Each individual's blood sugar journey is distinct. Regular monitoring grants you a personal window into how your body navigates different scenarios, enabling you to make decisions aligned with your unique needs.

Empowerment Through Knowledge: The data gleaned from monitoring empowers you to make informed choices. As you witness the impact of lifestyle factors on blood sugar, you become an active participant in your health journey.

Blood Sugar Patterns: The Blueprint of Wellness

Regular monitoring lays bare the intricate interplay between your choices and blood sugar levels. Here are some common patterns that monitoring can unveil:

Post-Meal Spikes: Tracking post-meal blood sugar levels reveals how certain foods influence your body's response. High-carbohydrate meals can lead to spikes, highlighting the need for mindful carb management.

Morning Readings: Morning blood sugar levels provide insight into your body's fasting response. Elevated morning readings might necessitate adjustments to bedtime snacks or medications.

Exercise Impact: Monitoring before and after exercise showcases how physical activity affects blood sugar. It also guides you in finding the optimal timing for activity to prevent spikes or crashes.

Stress Signals: Stress can impact blood sugar levels. By monitoring during stressful periods, you can identify stress-induced fluctuations and incorporate relaxation techniques.

Sleep Clues: Blood sugar levels during sleep hours can reveal the phenomenon of the "dawn effect," where glucose rises in the morning. This insight informs strategies to manage morning readings.

Nutrition Unveiled: A Data-Driven Approach

Regular monitoring aligns with the principle that knowledge is power. Armed with blood sugar data, you can shape your nutritional choices with precision, considering how different foods impact your levels.

Carbohydrate Awareness: Monitoring helps you identify the carbohydrates that prompt steep rises in blood sugar. Armed with this knowledge, you can choose low glycemic index options to prevent spikes.

Meal Timing: Timing your meals in relation to monitoring sessions can help you gauge the effects of different foods. This information guides you in creating balanced, satisfying meals.

Balancing Act: Monitoring fosters a balanced approach to eating. You can enjoy occasional treats while being aware of their impact on blood sugar.

Physical Activity Synergy: A Guiding Light

Monitoring blood sugar levels before and after exercise offers valuable insights into how physical activity interacts with your body's glucose response.

Pre-Activity Levels: Monitoring before exercise helps you understand your starting point. Lower blood sugar levels might require a light snack to prevent drops during activity.

Post-Activity Readings: Tracking post-exercise blood sugar levels reveals how your body responds to different types and durations of activity. This knowledge guides adjustments for future workouts.

Empowerment in Action: From Data to Lifestyle Mastery

"Keep track of blood sugar levels to identify patterns and adjust your lifestyle accordingly" encapsulates a journey of empowerment—a journey that transforms raw data into actionable insights. By embracing regular monitoring, you weave a narrative of control—one that resonates with informed decisions, precision in choices, and the ability to navigate the intricate dance of blood sugar regulation. Every entry in your monitoring log is a step in the symphony of your well-being—a step that echoes with empowerment, knowledge, and a life that is masterfully tuned.

Chapter <14>

Weight Management: Navigating the Path to Balance and Insulin Sensitivity

In the intricate canvas of health, weight management stands as a cornerstone—an artful journey that paints vitality through equilibrium. The chapter "Weight Management" beckons us to explore the art of achieving and maintaining a healthy weight, a voyage that transcends aesthetics to shape the canvas of insulin sensitivity. As we embark on this exploration, we'll unravel the profound interplay between weight, insulin resistance, and well-being, crafting a narrative of resilience, empowerment, and lasting health.

Weight's Role in Insulin Sensitivity: An Interwoven Narrative

The relationship between weight and insulin resistance is intricate, unveiling a tale of profound implications for metabolic harmony. Insulin resistance, characterised by reduced responsiveness to insulin, is a key driver of type 2 diabetes—a condition where blood sugar levels rise beyond optimal levels. Weight management becomes a compass in this narrative, guiding us toward reducing the risk of insulin resistance.

The Weight-Insulin Axis: Excess body weight, especially abdominal fat, contributes to insulin resistance. Adipose tissue, or fat cells, release hormones that hinder insulin's effectiveness, leading to higher blood sugar levels.

A Balancing Act: Achieving a healthy weight restores the equilibrium between insulin and glucose. A balanced body weight supports improved insulin sensitivity, enhancing the body's ability to regulate blood sugar.

Weight Loss and Insulin Sensitivity: The Empowering Connection

Weight loss, when approached mindfully and sustainably, can spark a cascade of benefits that rekindle insulin sensitivity and reduce the risk of diabetes.

Fat Cell Dynamics: Weight loss reduces the release of insulin-resistant hormones from fat cells, allowing insulin to function more effectively.

Glucose Uptake: Shedding excess weight enhances glucose uptake by cells, promoting stable blood sugar levels and reducing strain on the body's insulin production.

Strategies for Achieving and Sustaining a Healthy Weight

Embarking on a journey of weight management necessitates intention, patience, and balanced choices. Here are strategies to navigate this path with grace and efficacy:

Nutrition Wisdom: Adopt a balanced and nutritious eating plan that suits your preferences and lifestyle. Prioritise whole foods, vegetables, lean proteins, and complex carbohydrates.

Mindful Portions: Cultivate portion control to prevent overeating. Be attentive to your body's hunger and fullness cues, aiming for satisfaction without excess.

Regular Physical Activity: Engage in regular exercise that aligns with your fitness level and interests. Cardiovascular workouts, strength training, and flexibility exercises contribute to a holistic fitness routine.

Sustainable Lifestyle Changes: Embrace gradual, sustainable changes rather than quick fixes. Small adjustments in habits and routines can lead to lasting weight management.

Behavioural Awareness: Recognize emotional eating triggers and cultivate alternative coping strategies. Engaging in mindfulness, deep breathing, or engaging hobbies can redirect emotional impulses.

Hydration Habits: Stay hydrated, as thirst can sometimes be mistaken for hunger. Drinking water throughout the day supports balanced eating.

Professional Guidance: Consult with healthcare professionals, such as a registered dietitian or a fitness trainer, to create a tailored weight management plan that aligns with your health goals.

The Empowerment in Every Step: A Journey of Resilience

"Achieve and maintain a healthy weight to reduce the risk of insulin resistance" encapsulates a journey of empowerment—a journey that transcends numbers on a scale to evoke lasting health. By embracing the path of weight management, you craft a narrative of strength—one that resonates with balance, vitality, and a life that's attuned to well-being. Each choice you make, each step you take towards a healthy weight, is a brushstroke in the portrait of your health—a brushstroke that echoes with empowerment, knowledge, and a life that's beautifully aligned.

Chapter <15>

Medically Supervised Plans: Navigating Wellness Through Expert Guidance

In the intricate landscape of health, medically supervised plans stand as a beacon of wisdom—a path guided by the expertise of medical professionals. The chapter "Medically Supervised Plans" extends an invitation to explore the art of seeking personalised guidance, including medications and insulin therapy if necessary. This journey transcends self-direction, weaving a narrative of empowerment and tailored well-being. As we delve into this exploration, we'll unveil the profound impact of medical supervision on blood sugar management, revealing the harmony between expert guidance and individual health aspirations.

The Expertise of Medical Professionals: A Guiding Light

In the intricate dance of blood sugar regulation, the guidance of medical professionals is akin to a compass that illuminates the way. Expertise in diabetes management, medication usage, and insulin therapy empowers individuals to navigate the complexities of their health with precision and confidence.

Personalised Approach: Medical professionals craft a personalised roadmap, aligning interventions with your unique health profile, goals, and lifestyle. This tailored approach enhances the effectiveness of interventions.

Optimal Medication Usage: Medical supervision ensures that medications are administered optimally—addressing not only blood sugar control but also potential interactions, side effects, and adjustments.

Insulin Therapy Mastery: For individuals requiring insulin therapy, medical professionals provide invaluable guidance. They prescribe appropriate insulin types, dosages, and administration methods tailored to your needs.

The Medically Supervised Journey: An Empowering Narrative

Embracing medically supervised plans empowers individuals to take charge of their health journey with the support of expert knowledge. Here's how this journey unfolds:

Thorough Assessment: Medical professionals conduct a comprehensive assessment of your health, considering factors such as blood sugar levels, medical history, lifestyle, and goals.

Personalised Guidance: Based on the assessment, medical professionals develop a tailored plan that may include dietary recommendations, exercise regimens, medication adjustments, or insulin therapy.

Educational Empowerment: Medical supervision is accompanied by education—understanding how medications work, insulin administration techniques, and lifestyle adjustments that foster optimal blood sugar management.

Ongoing Monitoring: Regular appointments with medical professionals allow for ongoing assessment, adjustments, and discussions about progress, challenges, and changes in health status.

Collaborative Decision-Making: Medically supervised plans are characterised by collaboration between you and your healthcare team. Your input, concerns, and preferences play a pivotal role in shaping the trajectory of your plan.

Navigating Medications: A Strategic Approach

Medications play a vital role in blood sugar management for many individuals. Under the guidance of medical professionals, medications can be tailored to your needs for optimal efficacy:

Oral Medications: These medications can enhance insulin sensitivity, stimulate insulin production, or slow carbohydrate absorption. Medical supervision ensures their appropriate usage and potential adjustments.

Injectable Medications: In some cases, injectable medications other than insulin may be prescribed. Medical professionals guide you through their administration, dosages, and potential side effects.

Insulin Therapy: For individuals requiring insulin, medical supervision is paramount. Medical professionals determine the right insulin regimen, monitor its effectiveness, and provide education on insulin administration techniques.

The Role of Expert Knowledge: A Journey of Wellness

"Consult medical professionals for personalised guidance, including medications and insulin therapy if needed" encapsulates a journey of collaboration—a journey where your health aspirations are nurtured by the hands of experts. By embracing medically supervised plans, you craft a narrative of partnership—one that resonates with informed decisions, tailored interventions, and a life that's guided by expert knowledge. Each appointment, each consultation with your healthcare team, is a chapter in the story of your health—a chapter that echoes with empowerment, mastery, and a life that's harmoniously aligned.